Table of Contents

Introduction

As a man, you should know that there is one particular organ in your body that you should take special care of – the prostate. It is for your future, and to some extent, for the future of human kind that you give this part of your body some TLC. Personally, I never thought I would have to be so cautious about it. Now that I'm having problems with my own prostate, it's obvious that I should have paid more attention to what my body was trying to tell me through its signs and actions. I just neglected it. I'm afraid to say that over the past eight months the price I've been paying for the negligence is quite overwhelming. You may still have a chance of improving things in your situation. Read on and you'll find out what I've experienced during this time and what triggered the 'curse of the prostate' in my case. One more thing – if you're beginning to think that there is something wrong with your 'ejaculation organ', please be advised to see a doctor – it could be something trivial, or it could be something big and serious.

Oh, and let me set you straight on this – I'm not a dietician or a nutritionist, or a doctor. Just an average sort of guy who's got to know stuff by having been through things. If you find helpful the information contained in this e-book, then you've made me a happy man, genuinely :-)

Terms and conditions

No worries. It's not what you think. I've been reading a lot about bladder and, in particular, prostate problems in men, like prostatitis and prostate enlargement. Through trial and error, I've managed to improve some of the symptoms of my prostate, and so decided to get the stuff together and share it with you, possibly having the same trouble on your mind. I really hope the findings selected and collected in this publication will be of help to you, too.

But before that, here's a brief introduction to the terminology that is used and that you can encounter when having problems with the prostate gland:

- *bladder* – a bag-like organ where urine is stored. The bladder is located directly above the prostate.

- *rectum* – the lowest end of the bowels through which your poo comes out

- *prostate gland* (in short *prostate*) – it is located right beneath the bladder. Most people describe it as a walnut-shaped reproductive organ. The gland surrounds the urethra. That's why when you get older or when the prostate gets inflamed or infected it becomes bigger, at which point it can be really hard and painful for you to urinate.

- *urethra* – quite a long tube beginning at the bottom of the bladder, passing through the surrounding prostate gland and then through the penis, where it ends. It is this tube that carries your urine and semen out of your body. A male's urethra is on average 5 times as long as a female's.

- *benign prostatic hyperplasia* or *hypertrophy* (*BPH*, or commonly known and referred to as *prostate enlargement*) – a noncancerous (benign) enlargement of the prostate, a condition that affects around 50% of men aged 50 and over, and nearly 70-80% of those over the age of 70. It is caused by an increased growth of cells in the prostate. It can cause urinary problems, including urinary tract obstruction. It is not related to prostate cancer.

- *prostatitis* – an inflammation of the prostate, typically occurring in men under the age of 50 (accounting for up to 10%). It is often caused by bacteria, but many a time the cause is unknown. Some men may develop chronic prostatitis that keeps coming back again and again. Like BPH, it is not related to cancer but can cause urinary problems.

  There are four major types of prostatitis: (a) acute bacterial prostatitis; (b) chronic bacterial prostatitis; (c) chronic non-bacterial prostatitis (also known as *chronic pelvic pain syndrome* or *CPPS*; often referred to as *prostatodynia* or *prostadynia*); (d) asymptomatic inflammatory prostatitis.

- *prostate cancer* – a life-threatening condition of the prostate gland. The chances of developing prostate cancer increase as you get older. Most cases develop in men aged 50 or older. Bear in mind that symptoms associated with this type of cancer are similar to symptoms of other conditions that can affect the prostate. So it's best to see your GP to get them right.

- *digital rectal examination* (*DRE*) – this is when the doctor sticks his or her finger into your rectum to check for any abnormalities of your prostate – don't worry, the doctor is wearing a glove that is usually lubricated during the examination, so it's not that bad or painful

- *void* – as a noun, a medical term for the discharge of the contents of the bowels or bladder; and as a verb, the meaning is *to excrete*. In this case, however, take it as another term for an act of *urination* and *to urinate*, respectively.

I'm afraid you'll have to try the Internet for more information on any of those and other related subjects.

The all-important symptoms

The following most typical symptoms can indicate possible problems with your bladder or prostate:

- painful lower back, especially when you get up in the morning and you wouldn't expect a pain in that part of your body, because you know you didn't work out hard the day before

- dribbling or no ability to push out the last few drops of urine at the end of void

- when urinating, the stream stops and starts again several times

- weak or too strong a flow

- constipation or an attack of diarrhoea

- dark-coloured urine, or blood in your urine that can make it go dark

- feeling of needing to urinate frequently during the night

- feeling of needing to urinate urgently during the day

- difficulty keeping the urine in the bladder

Any of the symptoms could actually indicate that there is a problem in your body, not particularly with your bladder or prostate, but I had most of them when I was first struck with a bladder infection, so I assume they're most relevant.

What the heck is going on?

Ok. Here's a long story of mine cut short. Back in February 2014, I got a nasty bladder infection. It wasn't until two weeks after the first symptoms that I found out what it actually was. Exactly on the eve of my birthday, I woke up, did my bit in the toilet – well, two bits, to be precise – and then had a dreadful shock. My penis got so small, virtually the size of your pinkie, that I got into panic. I thought I'd never be able to urinate again! It got that small and extremely stiff. I couldn't pull back the foreskin at all, which was another concern – normally, you can do it without a problem unless you're already suffering from *phimosis* – that's when the front of your foreskin is tight and narrow, and you cannot retract it without making damage to it, like painful splits in the skin. Well, to be honest with you, I had already been suffering from the condition back then. I could, however, get the foreskin move backwards a bit so that I could clean it from time to time.

So, what happened next. I got back to my room upstairs. I was so frightened that I decided to get myself to A&E straight away. I hardly ever visit a doctor. What's more, I still don't have a GP. I just feel that when I am taken ill, first of all, I try to sort things out with my own initiative. You know, some over-the-counter medicine would normally deal with any problem I had. But not this time.

Oh, I would've forgotten to mention one more thing – the night before my legs and feet had become very swollen. To my horror, my shoes didn't fit any more. And when I took my socks off before going to bed, I noticed that the skin of my calves, and especially of my shins, took the shape of the socks. I mean, the depression left on my legs after taking the socks off was extremely noticeable. Even keeping my feet up couldn't help with getting my legs and feet as they were before – skinny and bony.

That was two weeks after the initial symptoms. 'Why did it take you a fortnight to eventually see a doctor?' you might be asking. Well, like I said, I try my own methods first. The problem began with a smelly penis. And I mean an extremely smelly penis. At that point, I thought I'd give it a wash and that would be it. But when I got under the foreskin, I could see some sticky, whitish stuff covering my glans. I washed it off my penis only to discover that it was inflamed – I mean red in colour. At first, I thought it was just a change of colour in my penis. Nothing serious to worry about. And I carried on with my life as normal.

After two days, my penis got itchy to the point that I just had to scratch it more and more. That must have caused even more inflammation. I began to clean it every day. But the redness wouldn't go. After another five days, things got really worse. I had just taken a hot bath when I started to feel 'itchy inside my bladder'. I mean, I couldn't resist moving my legs and pelvis to stop the uncomfortable feeling. I was sort of squeezing the muscles of my bladder to stop the feeling, as if trying to pull back the urine that was already inside my bladder. The worst thing came when I began to feel an extreme urge for urinating. That was as nasty as it gets. I couldn't overcome it in any way. I had to go to the toilet every hour or so. And that persisted for another week. Day and night. I was getting more and more exhausted. I googled some stuff and it became obvious to me that I was suffering from a *UTI*, that is a *urinary tract infection*. It was advisable to drink plenty of fluid, which I did and which made me visit the toilet even more frequently. Nights were never the same any more. I couldn't keep the urine in my bladder for long periods of time. Sometimes, it was just a few drops of urine that made me rush to the toilet!

I couldn't go on like this, but I am a stubborn person. I started taking supplements of vitamin C to make my urine acidic, which apparently makes flushing the bacteria more easily. I started drinking herbal teas, like chamomile and nettle, which can supposedly fight off infections. And to be honest with you, I was beginning to feel better and better. But that was all to no avail. I ended up seeing a doctor anyway.

Have you been feeling run-down recently?

That's what the doctor said after it turned out that I was struggling with a UTI. Apart from the infection I was diagnosed with, I also had a temperature. A week-long course of antibiotics, TRIMETHOPRIM 200mg, would do me good, the doctor continued. As for the stiffness of my penis at that time, he couldn't say what it was. But it seemed to me that the infection was so severe that it had caused my penis to shrink and retract into the pelvis. Luckily, after a day the things regarding my penis got back to normal. Unlike my bladder, which was still making my life unbearable.

The common question

Was it because I neglected my infection that I've been suffering from a bad prostate? Or was it my prostate I never took much notice of that actually caused the infection? I haven't a clue. It's like asking, 'Which came first: the chicken or the egg?' The thing is, I had my prostate checked out by doctors while I visited my family for Easter in 2014. Two samples of my urine and semen were collected and tested for bacteria. None were found in either of the samples. So I was clear, as far as bacteria were concerned. But I still had this nagging feeling of needing to urinate. The ultrasound scan of my bladder revealed that there was no urine retention. My prostate, I mean the size of it, was normal. The doctor pointed out that it could be something to do with the nervous system that was somehow affected by the infection. He meant to prescribe me some tablets for the so-called 'overactive bladder', but eventually decided against it. He did, however, prescribe me some other antibiotics. It was just a two-day course. I couldn't tell any difference after taking them whether I got better or worse. I just followed the doctor's orders.

So, by the beginning of summer I could say that I had been cured of the UTI. Don't get me wrong, though. The first course of antibiotics did the trick. They killed the bacteria and effectively stopped them from spreading further. I just felt that there was still something inside my bladder that was making me feel uncomfortable. The feeling of my prostate as if being enlarged was still a problem to me up till December 2014.

I strongly believe that there's always an issue with the prostate gland after suffering from a bladder infection. They just feel as one to me, one organ going through the other. Whatever fluids you produce in your body will gather in your bladder. Your semen will use the same route out as your urine does – through the urethra and penis. Also, problems with your prostate will, in most cases, affect your bladder. So once you've developed a condition with either of the two, you can expect to suffer from both. This, at least, seems to have been the case with me.

(What follows is updated information that I put in this e-book after initial

Later in 2014, when I was visiting my family – this time for Christmas – I went to see a doctor to have a routine check-up of my penis – I thought my prostate was fine then so I didn't ask for a DRE. And what happened? I got a massive blow! With a swab taken of my penis, I tested positive for… E coli (in full Escherichia coli), one of the most vicious bacteria that can cause serious illness or even death. It's ok to have them in your gut, but if they get somewhere else out, like your bladder – or in my case, penis – you're in for trouble. This was it! The bacterium was still in my system, making me feel uncomfortable with my prostate and bladder. My guts were forever telling me there was still something not right. And there was the culprit, E coli. I reckon the same E coli were initially responsible for my UTI back in February 2014.

This time I was prescribed with a course of antibiotics taken orally for 10 long days – there were two different kinds of antibiotic in a single tablet, supposedly working in synergy. Besides these, two different types of cream for regular application on the skin of my glans, up to four weeks. In a case that they wouldn't work, I was advised to see my doctor again. Four different antibiotics in total for the whole Christmas and more, including the New Year. I felt horrible throughout the treatment. I was weak and lacking energy to do anything. I was miserable all the time. At least, I kept alive the hope that the medication for the bacteria might finally clear them up.

It's 2015 when I'm writing this. Towards the end of January. I feel good, although there is still a patchy piece of skin on my glans. It looks to me like the bacteria are back, but I'm applying some colloidal silver cream – instead of the antibiotic creams I was previously prescribed – and it feels all right. My bladder is 'calm'. I mean it doesn't make me feel uncomfortable, as was the case before when it felt like it was not fully emptied after a visit to the loo. My prostate feels good, too. There's no feeling of a ball stuck between my buttocks any more. So at least, these symptoms are gone. I can freely ride my bicycle again! Hopefully, the colloidal silver cream will do the trick. If not, I've still got those creams packed full of antibiotics, I might have to start using them again.

It's still 2015 now, the very beginning of October. I feel absolutely great having spent a wonderful time with my family back in my home country, Poland.

During that time, I was involved in a lot of physical activities. My body had to work hard as it used to. It wasn't just visiting my family; rather, I wanted to make my body sweat like hell. The magnificent weather helped with that to a massive extent. It was scorching hot for long periods of summertime.

Why am I writing about this? I thought I was able to get some fat off my belly (yep, when I got back to my English home I had lost eight pounds of my body weight and the 'bump' on my belly), which I believe had significantly contributed to my prostate symptoms improved. The weight of that bump must have had an impact on how my guts, and especially my bladder and prostate gland, were continually squashed by the weight of all the fat I had before. No such feeling as if I had a tennis ball stuck in between my buttocks!

There is also one thing I am certain about that helped me too – the psychological thing. Before, I felt depressed and unwilling to take part in any activities whatsoever. Now I feel as though I could carry mountains ☺. I am all in favour of the idea that 'it all starts here, in your mind'. The better I feel, the less trouble I am having with my prostate and bladder problems. That's what I do believe was the case with me.

Oh, I would have forgotten to mention this – I'm on a course of some herbal medicine, soft tranquilizers including valerian and cistus incanus, which are doing a great job with my stress-laden life. I feel more relaxed and sleep better than before. I'd recommend such to you as well. What can I say, happy days again in my life!

(End of updated information)

Dos and don'ts

And here we are. The information and recommendations that follow have all been put to the test by myself. I know what has helped me most and what hasn't agreed with my prostate. Bear in mind that it's a personal thing how your body reacts to things. So if you find that something recommended here is no good for you, or you already know that, please don't even try it.

Physical activity

Walking and running

Lack of exercise can make you ill. Spending too much time within the walls of your bedroom can also make you ill. I mean it's not the room by itself that is so bad, but the stale air hanging in it. You need oxygen to allow your body to function properly. Your prostate is almost stagnant. The blood doesn't circulate in it as lively as in other parts of your body, and consequently, lack of oxygen in your prostate can make it feel ill too. Running, and especially, walking is highly recommended. The movement of your legs is like a massage – your prostate gets a soft stroke with every single step you take. Since every organ is covered in millions of nerves, the stimulation of the prostate gland can alleviate any pain in it. As if by magic, physical activity can really improve the comfort of your life. Well, it surely has to me.

Sitting and lying down

Try not to sit for longer periods of time. If you have to spend a lot of time sitting, try standing up and walking around the place where you are as often as every half an hour. Believe it or not, but sitting has a massive impact on the gland. You must realize that you're actually sitting on your prostate. It gets squeezed by the upper organs, like the stomach, bowels and bladder every time you take the position of the capital letter 'L'. Besides, the nerves that connect your bladder to the brain through carrying the signals also get squeezed and may become permanently 'mangled', just like the cables of your earphones when you take them out of your pocket after being stuck and kept in it for a long time.

On the one hand, lying down is all right. It doesn't have such a negative effect on the prostate as sitting does. Putting your body in horizontal position is like taking weight off your chest, or speaking in a psychological fashion, taking a load off your mind. But here, it's not the chest or mind that takes advantage of such a move, it's your prostate, obviously. Give it a rest as you would to your whole body.

On the other hand, when you're already struggling with your bladder, changing position from horizontal to vertical can also have an impact on the gland. It's got something to do with the muscles of your legs and the muscles of the floor of your pelvic. This seems to have been the case with me. Once I feel that I need to do a wee, my penis swells with muscle tension and this makes it harder for me to urinate. The swelling has always left me with the feeling that my bladder hasn't emptied fully following the wee. Feeling wet at the tip of your penis and actually leaving the 'last drop' on your underwear after urinating is also typical of this condition. The more obstructed the route to the urethra, the more difficult it is for you to void. This can cause your kidneys to work less effectively and eventually lead to kidney failure. This is because the possible obstruction around the top of your urethra and the bottom of your bladder – the place where they meet – can make the pressure pushing the urine out of the bladder damage your kidneys through the so-called 'reverse or back flow'. I've been able to somehow improve on this by sitting on the toilet instead of standing and leaning over it. The muscles feel much more relaxed when sitting down.

There is also another trick that has been working for me – once I'm standing up, I move about for a while, like a minute, and then sit down for another minute, or for as long as it takes for me to feel that my penis has shrunk, and then I'm off to the loo. It appears to me that the trick helps with relieving the tension of the muscles surrounding the prostate and bladder.

Cycling

I used to love cycling. Even now I tend to get around my town on my pushbike more often than on any other means of transport. But the problems concerning my prostate have made me more reluctant to do so. It hurts. Every time I get on and off the saddle, my penis enlarges to the point that the tip of it, I mean the glans, leaves the foreskin zone, as if pushed forward by the prostate. I think the pressure on the prostate while sitting on a bike is even greater than when sitting in a chair. Any uneven surface on the road or pavement that I have to go over hits back my pelvis and surely makes my prostate feel it as hard as well. Nowadays, I tend to stand up on the pedals every time I get to a curb or anything that is higher or lower than the surface I am riding on. Honestly, cycling is no joy to me anymore. I'm thinking of buying myself a saddle that is not stiff – one that is supported on springs – which should take the impact of any bumps on my way and improve the overall experience.

Intercourse and masturbation

Having sex is a real joy. But everything changes when you suffer from a troubled prostate. It is claimed that when you have sex, you release all the tension in the prostate gland and thus making it shrink to the point that it stops putting a pressure on the bladder and urethra. It is advisable that you empty your bladder after every single intercourse you have. So, basically you should be as sexually active as possible. That's what people say. I, however, beg to differ a bit on this issue. It surely helps in some way. But you must realise that any flexible organ that is 'flushed' will fill up again with fluid eventually. It so happens that an enlarged prostate tends to grow towards the inside of it rather than the outside. This will cause a narrowing of the urethra and therefore you won't be able to pass urine easily. You can tell that your passageway has shrunk by the pressure of your stream. An archy stream is supposed to be good, whereas a straight one is not. My stream tended to be straight in the morning and evening, and looked archy during the day. But since I started to sit on the toilet while having a pee , I can't actually tell what it is like now. At least, I feel more comfortable than before when standing.

The same goes for masturbation. The more you do it, the more it feels like it's helping you. But it's not. What you really need is something that would make your prostate flush and get rid of any bad stuff that will normally collect in it. The solution is – the prostate massage.

The 'mighty' prostate massage

It is absolutely not the same as intercourse or masturbation, as most people think. The prostate massage consists in releasing the tension of the prostate gland, which in effect makes the gland clean itself of the debris that collects in the prostate after a period of time, and especially when you're sexually inactive. When you have sex and you come, your semen is released together with other fluids that act as sperm carriers. Only a bit of the bad stuff gets its way out of the prostate during that process. Women have antibodies in their wombs that can easily fight any bad guys coming from a man's penis. This, together with the fact that there is more good stuff than bad stuff coming through when having sex or playing with yourself, should make you aware of the two different ways that your prostate actually works. The outcome of the prostate massage is more 'filthy', so to speak.

Your doctor can perform a massage on your prostate to collect samples of the fluids that the prostate gland produces. This is often done to check out for any infection that can be present in the organ. In the past, it used to be an effective method of curing defective prostates, especially enlarged ones. Such practice seems to have been abandoned due to the fact that it would normally take more than one massage to actually work its magic. It just takes too much time for a doctor to treat one patient with the condition. Besides, any problems with your prostate that you may have had in the past tend to recur in the future. I'm afraid the same applies to any UTIs. Once you've suffered from one, expect another to happen again one day. Like a boomerang, it will return. You're doomed to have one back over and over again.

There are some tips on the Web on how to perform a prostate massage on your own, but to my way of thinking and understanding, it's not easy to do it at all. I personally wouldn't recommend it.

Wet dream, or nocturnal emission

This is the magic wand, as it were. It's quite embarrassing to wake up with your pants wet. But believe me, and I'm telling you this from first-hand experience, that there is no need to feel that way. This is the natural gift that we were given by the Creator himself. It so happens that in my mother tongue, Polish, the medical term for this is 'polucja' (from Latin 'pollutio' or 'pollutionis', which means *pollution* in English). The word itself perfectly reflects the whole phenomenon.

Too much of something is never good for you. Your prostate constantly produces sperm. All the excess and unused sperm, often dead sperm cells – what I call the bad stuff or 'debris' – must somehow go out of your system. This also happens, you might not know, when you urinate. But the most natural and effective way of getting rid of the bad stuff is by wet dream. This will clean your prostate as well as the doctor would with his or her finger when performing a prostate massage. In the case of a wet dream, the ratio of the sperm and the bad stuff nearly equals. It is through this performance of your prostate that you can actually feel any improvement that I strongly feel is worth writing about. Wet dreams more often occur in men who stay sexually inactive for longer periods of time than in those sexually active. I hadn't had a wet dream until three weeks ago, for over six months. But I used to experience them quite often, on a regular basis. Actually, I can tell that the lack of wet dreams had something to do with my initial problems with the bladder. The infection had kind of shut this almost miraculous capability of the prostate completely down. Read on to find out what caused one to happen to me again after such a long time (just to remind you, six months).

So my personal advice would be that you try living in celibacy for a while. A bit of a sacrifice, I know. Basically, stay away from any sexual activity for as long as you finally get a wet dream. In my case, it was a huge relief when I got it. At first, when I woke up in the middle of the night, I dreaded that my prostate had burst, which you should know might happen, especially in cases when the gland is seriously enlarged and severely inflamed. I had a temperature and my heartbeat got irregular with palpitations. I'm sure I panicked. I felt extremely ill. No wonder I felt that way, I had been waiting for a wet dream for so long that it felt like a volcano eruption, surely not like a simple ejaculation. To my surprise and delight, another wet dream occurred a few days soon after. This one was more comfortable. The weird thing was that, unlike I remembered it previously when I was getting it regularly, I had no recollection of sexuality-laden dream, which is typical in these circumstances. Nothing whatsoever. Well, I didn't care much about it. I was quite happy that I had experienced it once again.

It's been a while since I last had those wet dreams. I'm definitely feeling better than before them. I'm looking forward to another one, since the sensation of my bladder not being emptied fully is still the issue. At least, riding my bike feels more comfortable again. Even sitting in front of the computer, which is the case right at this moment in time, feels comfy and there is none of this feeling as if I was sitting on a tennis ball. Happy days, really.

One more thing, you would have thought it's easy to make wet dreams occur if and whenever you wanted them to. But that's just not true. It's a natural thing. I don't know of any techniques or methods that could bring about wet dreams just like that. So patience is key here.

As a side note – I may be wrong or it was just a coincidence, but the two separate wet dreams I experienced happened when I had taken a tablespoonful of pumpkin seed oil the night before, just a couple of hours before going to bed. So I think it's well worth trying this out.

Food and drink

Tomatoes

Right, this is a bit tricky. Most of the reviews and opinions I came across on the Net about tomatoes and their impact on the prostate were positive. I mean, doctors and people affected by prostate problems recommended eating tomatoes because of their beneficial properties. In any form, but the more the tomatoes were processed in the heat, the more recommended they were. Like tomato paste, which was my first choice when I started feeding myself on it. At least one study that I remember suggested taking up to 50g of the paste per day for up to 12 weeks or so. It had shown that by doing so the enlarged prostate would shrink, which was the case in over 70% in men taking the challenge in the study. Basically, likopen – the key helping factor in red tomatoes and, in fact, in any other vegetables of similar colour – is claimed to protect against cancer.

So, I thought to myself, 'Why not try.' And so I did try but had to stop. I was at week 7, I think. It felt that my prostate was suffering from too much of the stuff. The feeling of enlargement in the pelvic area was becoming insufferable. At this point, I recollected reading this article saying that eating tomatoes was not recommended at all when experiencing problems with the prostate. That was based on a German research the results of which had shown that tomatoes weren't that good for the gland as most other sources would suggest. I believe this must be an individual case. Your prostate may be more tolerant than mine. Tomatoes are well worth trying in the treatment of any prostatic issues.

Garlic

Two important minerals to your prostate, that is zinc and selenium, can both be found in garlic. However, garlic can give you wind, which in effect can make you feel bloated on your belly. And that extra stress may have a negative impact on your prostate. It may get irritated by the movement of wind in the bowels.

Personally, I eat a few cloves of garlic every day. Not raw, as I used to. I put them in my soups when making them. This kills the harsh taste and makes it less strong to your tongue. However, the trick makes the garlic less effective – it just loses its most potent ingredient, allicin, responsible for garlic's anti-bacterial and anti-fungal properties. But I'm quite sure the minerals don't get depleted in their amounts in the heating process, so I reckon it's fine to do so. My advice to you would be that if you eat garlic and you start feeling bad, just give it a miss then. You should be fine with the other recommended stuff.

Cranberries

The berries of North America, what I personally like to call them, are good in preventing UTIs both in men and women. I know nothing of them as being of any benefit to the prostate, though. Telling you from my own experience, I can say that they do what they're claimed to. I wish I had known what I know now about cranberries when I first caught a UTI. I might have not fallen ill if I had been eating cranberries in the first place. Bear in mind that they can't cure you of infections in your bladder. They just prevent them, or help fight them more effectively when you have one. If you didn't fancy increasing your daily sugar intake ('cause cranberries contain a lot of it), or especially when you're diabetic, go for cranberry extract supplements. Otherwise, feel free to drink as much cranberry juice as you like. Snacking on dried cranberries is also good (watch out for your teeth, though). In my case, once I stop taking the supplements, the infection will return instantly. I mean the frequency when I need to go to the loo will increase dramatically. So I know exactly what is going on again. It may be a mental thing, but I now try not to skip any tablets. Remember that the sooner you take action when you feel ill, the better your chances of eradicating the infection at its early stage. Act immediately to stop it at its core.

Quercetin

What is it, this quercetin? Well, it belongs to a group of plant pigments known as *bioflavonoids*. And bioflavonoids, or flavonoids in short (from Latin 'flavus' meaning *yellow*), are basically naturally occurring pigments that some laboratory studies have indicated may have potential anti-cancer properties, but usually only when consumed in large quantities. You can find quercetin in many citrus fruits, but I've been taking supplements which contain more of the stuff than the average fruit does. I think it has helped improve some of the symptoms of my bad prostate. As long as it doesn't make my symptoms get worse, I feel all right taking it with my food. If my memory serves me right, the recommended daily allowance of quercetin is 500mg.

Pumpkin seed oil

I strongly believe that this, together with lots of magnesium in my diet, has helped me most. I mean, extremely most! Funnily enough, I ordered a couple of pumpkin seed oil only after seeing the BBC series, *Hairy Bikers' Bakeation*. You know, I'm talking about the two entertaining guys, Si King and Dave Myers, travelling on their motorbikes and tasting the best baking on offer on their way across Europe. They were in Austria when I learnt that pumpkin seed oil was good for your prostate. Surprisingly, the stuff that I subsequently bought came from an Austrian farm dealing with pumpkin seeds only. Roasted seeds in this case. They basically grew the pumpkins merely to take the seeds out of the pumpkins and then make a delicious oil out of them.

Here's the most important bit about the oil and magnesium – after just two weeks of taking both of them, I finally experienced my long-awaited wet dream. You can't know how happy I was when it happened to me. I don't think there was anything else that might have contributed to this. It was at that very time that I was taking the oil and magnesium on a daily basis. A tablespoonful of pumpkin seed oil per day seemed to be sufficient, as it has ever since. It is now one of my everyday foods I regard as important to the prostate as water to the whole body. I think that taking the oil a couple of hours before bedtime is more effective. For me, it's like a potion keeping me alive and kicking. Seriously. The improvement on my prostate has been dramatic. I no longer need to get up at night and rush to the toilet. I no longer have the feeling of a tennis ball stuck in my bottom. My penis doesn't get as big as it would before when standing up before going for a wee. I just feel that the flow I get in the toilet is much smoother than ever. I just cannot recommend the pumpkin seed oil more. See for yourself if it helps you too.

Oh, one more thing – eating pumpkin seeds or the oil itself can help you stay bug free, as they say.

Avocado seeds

Let my voice be heard by doctors and scientists – my strong intuition tells me that there is something very powerful and valuable about avocado seeds with regard to treating bad prostates. I tend to have this phenomenal capacity of seeing, hearing and feeling things that you can't normally see, hear or feel.

On a sunny spring day, I kind of felt in need of having an avocado. A mere whim to eat one. I got two. I ate the two, but couldn't say I liked the taste of them. I normally don't buy this fruit. What I really felt inside of me was something, like an inner voice, telling me to buy them not for their flesh, but... for their seeds. That's it. I followed the voice and put the seeds away on a shelf so that they would dry out. Later, I completely forgot about them.

When the winter came, I was doing some cleaning in my bedroom when I remembered them. I was on the point of throwing the seeds away, but again, the moment I touched them, my inner voice told me not to dispose of them just like that. I know it may sound ridiculous to you, like I was a nutter or something, but please believe me, I've got this kind of feeling haunting me at times that I now regard it as normal. I could say it's my 'sixth sense'. Surprisingly, after these few months when I decided to keep the seeds, I found some information on the Net that proved my inner voice kind of right. There was an article dealing with avocado seeds saying that they may have anti-tumour properties! Wow! In that case, if my intuition was telling me so firmly not to get rid of the seeds, I should do something with them. Frankly speaking, I still keep them in the same place. You know, my stomach is fairly sensitive and it doesn't always agree with the foods I eat. I'm a bit afraid of becoming sick. But I know that one day I'm going to grate it into my soup and eat it, just to see what impact it may have on my prostate. I just wish there was more evidence to prove my feeling completely right about these avocado seeds. There must be something special about them. I feel absolutely certain about it. Just need some more concrete, scientific proof to confirm it. That's all I'm asking... So, if you happen to be a doctor, or better still, a natural science researcher, could you please possibly pass my request on to people who might investigate further on this? Thank you so much in advance. And I really mean it.

Sugar, salt and fat

I strongly discourage you from consuming too much sugar when suffering from a bladder infection. The bacteria responsible for the condition loves 'sugary' environment, that is alkaline environment. They thrive on sugar. The more sugar in your bloodstream, the more difficult it will be for you to combat the infection. Rather, take a more responsible approach and, say, eat fruit that is sour. I would also suggest taking more vitamin C alongside quercetin. This is all to make your urine 'taste' acidic, which the bacteria hate. It might be a bit difficult for people already struggling with too much acid produced in their stomach, but once you start feeling better, you'll see my point. You know what they say, 'There's no gain without pain'. Bear in mind, however, that the optimum balance between 'sweet and sour' stuff in your system is key once you've fought off an infection.

As far as the prostate is concerned, I don't actually know what impact sugar, salt or fat may have on the gland. Some say that cutting down on all of these is also beneficial. As I've been advised not to take too much sugar in my diet (because of the recurring bladder infections) I assume that less sugar in your diet is definitely better. The same goes for salt and fat, which I tend to consume in moderation.

Herbal teas

For your bad bladder, I'd recommend drinking lots of chamomile and nettle tea. They help with flushing the toxins out of your system. There's also one more herb that, when I was ill, I drank in combination with the two types of tea mentioned earlier – dandelion. These all have a favourable impact on your kidneys, which work their nephrons out every time you suffer from an infection.

For your bad prostate, there is only one herb that I feel is worth mentioning. It's called *Epilobium parviflorum*, commonly known as *Smallflower Hairy Willowherb*. In actual fact, for example in Austria, it is regarded as medicine and often prescribed to men with their bad prostate. I myself was taking a tincture composed of alcohol and this herb when fighting my UTI. I haven't tried the tea, yet. I am going to get myself some, though. The more I read about the herb, the more I want to include it in my personal daily list of helping foods and drinks.

Probiotics

I've just started another course of highly-potent probiotics, 40 billion in one capsule. I don't know why but when I was having a battle with my UTI, I didn't take any probiotics. But I now remember taking them regularly a couple of years ago, and the results I was getting back then were very satisfying. There were long periods of time when I was feeling much better in general. I was getting less tired and more eager to get up to work. My digestion got better as well, meaning the constant bloat after eating heavy foods was gone. So I've decided to give them a try again. They're already claimed to possess health benefits. What the heck. If they're not doing any harm to my prostate, I'll stick to them.

And of course if you are on any antibiotics prescribed by your doctor for an infection, you should seriously consider taking probiotics while 'doing the course' and some time afterwards. They'll protect your good bacteria against the bad impact antibiotics usually have on the lining of your gut.

Colloidal silver

Another thing I've recently started taking on a regular basis is colloidal silver. It seems to be doing some good stuff to me – overall, I'm feeling quite well these days. Maybe it's me, thinking about my life in a more positive way, or it's the silver. Either way, I'd recommend trying it out. There's so much positive and generous feedback on colloidal silver that I genuinely thought I couldn't give it a miss. It's a really potent solution to many health problems you may have with your body. Before the era of antibiotics, colloidal silver ruled the world in that respect and was commonly prescribed by doctors.

The silver is claimed to be able to kill over 650 different strains of bacteria and viruses, without considerable side effects – as opposed to antibiotics, which can be really dangerous to you. One of the few side effects it may have is a condition called *argyria*. It occurs when silver builds up in the body – through prolonged contact with, or ingestion of, silver. It causes the skin to become blue or bluish-grey coloured. It is thought to be irreversible. Believe it or not, but it would take a lot of silver to be consumed for you to become affected by the condition. It's almost impossible to get it from just taking a couple of teaspoonfuls a day. You might always have a break in consumption after taking the silver for longer periods of time.

All in all, after pumpkin seed oil, vitamin D and magnesium, colloidal silver is another good thing to go for. It may take some time before you actually start seeing any positive changes in your wellbeing, but that's the case with everything, I believe. Just give it a go and see what it does to you.

Vitamins and minerals

Vitamin C

I've found that this vitamin is particularly helpful with bladder infections. Not alone, but combined with other things, like cranberries and quercetin. Besides, vitamin C can protect you from colds, which can make your body more susceptible to an infection. So obviously including enough fruit and vegetables in your everyday diet should be a wise move. My personal advice would be to take vitamin C supplements only when needed.

RDA (which stands for Recommended Daily Allowance) for vitamin C is 80mg per day (that is eighty milligrams). When being ill, it is suggested that you take up to 10 times as much. In the case when you suffer from too much acid in your stomach, you might opt for vitamin C supplementation in a non-acidic form like calcium ascorbate, making it gentle on your digestive system. And most importantly, be careful not to overdose on vitamin C.

Common foods high in vitamin C (milligrams – mg – per 100g):

- sweet peppers (180mg = 225% RDA)
- kiwis (92mg = 115% RDA)
- broccoli (90mg = 112% RDA)
- strawberries (60mg = 75% RDA)
- other berry fruits (on average 20-40mg = 25-50% RDA)
- green peas (58mg = 72% RDA)
- oranges (53mg = 66% RDA)
- other citrus fruits (on average 15-60mg = 20-75% RDA)
- tomatoes (23mg = 29% RDA)
- spinach (17mg = 21% RDA)

When taking supplements, especially, bear in mind that vitamin C is water soluble, meaning you need to drink fluid to absorb it.

Vitamin D

Did you know that your problems with the prostate, and bladder in particular, could stem from a lack of vitamin D in your system? The so-called 'sunshine vitamin' seems to play a massive role in the proper functioning of the two organs. The more vitamin D you get, like through exposing the skin of your body to sunlight, the more you benefit from it. Come winter and the need for the vitamin gets even more significant. Take my advice – spend as much time as you can outdoors in the summertime so that your body can store as much of vitamin D as it possibly can. Scientists say that 15 to 25 minutes spent in the sunshine daily should be enough for your body to be able to store sufficient amounts of sunshine vitamin for the coming winter. The best time to soak up the sun is between mid-April and mid-October, and then between 11am and 5pm. It's at that time that the sun is strongest. So if you're working night shifts, you should even try harder. I've heard that eating fatty fish, like mackerel, or taking fish liver oil supplements is a good way of supplying your body with this vitamin during the time when there's not much sunshine outside. As far as vitamin D supplements are concerned, I can't say much about them. It's true that I take them, but it's hard for me to give you any comments on them at the moment. I know from experience that the more time I spent in the sun, the better I felt with my prostate.

I remember it clearly that my UTI began in the wintertime. And it so happened that the previous year I had spent most of my time indoors, working on the computer. To my way of thinking, this kind of proves that vitamin D is important to your body, especially to your bladder. So I'd strongly advise you to do yourself a big favour and get enough of the vitamin, for goodness' sake.

RDA for vitamin D (as D3) is 5µg (or 5mcg – that is five micrograms) per day, or 200 IU (which stands for International Units; 40 IU = 1µg). Be particularly careful not to overdose on vitamin D – the toxicity threshold for vitamin D is thought to be between 250 and 1000µg per day (or between 10,000 and 40,000 IU). Only when prescribed by your doctor ought you to take high amounts of vitamin D.

Common foods high in vitamin D (micrograms – µg or mcg – per 100g):

- cod liver oil (250µg = 5000% RDA; per teaspoonful (5g) = 10µg = 200% RDA)
- oily fish, like mackerel (10µg = 200% RDA)
- vitamin D fortified cereals (5µg = 100% RDA)
- tofu (3.75µg = 75% RDA)
- butter (3.75µg = 75% RDA)
- eggs (2.5µg = 50% RDA)
- pork, like pork sausages or ham (2.5µg = 50% RDA)
- lard (2.5µg = 50% RDA)
- whole milk (1µg = 20% RDA)
- other dairy products, like yoghurt (on average 0.5 to 2µg = 10-40% RDA)

When taking supplements bear in mind that vitamin D is oil soluble, meaning you need to eat fat to absorb it.

Magnesium

This mineral is responsible for making you feel calmer. It's got a soothing effect on your nerves and muscles. I for one believe that it's in your mind that everything starts. So if you can, to some extent, control your mind, you'll be more capable of battling any troubles of your mind and body when you supply your system with magnesium. It's not easily absorbed from the foods you eat so going for supplements would also be recommended.

In my case, magnesium has massively contributed to how I've been managing to control my reactions to the stimuli of the world surrounding me. I am more than often stressed out. That's in my blood. And I know that the more nervous I get, the more I suffer. Together with the pumpkin seed oil and vitamin D, magnesium is the ideal solution for my prostate. They all work in the perfect synergy. It's like calling 'Bingo!' at a bingo gala. No more waiting for better results, as the ones I've got are sufficient to enhance my general well-being. I realise that the problems with my prostate may never disappear completely, but at least I feel I can carry on with my life again! The three easily available ingredients have made such an improvement on my physical and mental health that I could swear by them – they truly play a significant role in the processes that the prostate gland has to go under every day of your life. Try, as I have, implementing these in your life and you'll see for yourself. I just couldn't recommend them more to you, buddy. I honestly could not.

RDA for magnesium is 400mg per day. You should also be careful not to overdose on magnesium, as it could cause severe diarrhoea.

Common foods high in magnesium (milligrams –mg – per 100g):

- pumpkin seeds or pumpkin seed oil (534mg = 134% RDA)

- cocoa powder (500mg = 125% RDA)

- dark chocolate (330mg = 82% RDA)

- buckwheat (232mg = 58% RDA)

- other seeds, like sesame seeds (200mg = 50% RDA)

- almonds (180mg = 45% RDA)

- cashews (160mg = 40% RDA)

- peanuts or peanut butter (156mg = 39% RDA)

- fish, like mackerel (80mg = 20% RDA)

- spinach (80mg = 20% RDA)

- other nuts, like walnuts (60mg = 15% RDA)

- beans and lentils (60mg = 15% RDA)

- brown rice (44mg = 11% RDA)

- low-fat dairy products, like yoghurt (on average up to 40mg = 10% RDA)

- avocados (29mg = 7% RDA)

- bananas (27mg = 7% RDA)

- whole wheat pasta (27mg = 7% RDA)

Bear in mind that your body absorbs up to 50% of magnesium from the digestive system. To optimise the absorption, you should eat foods containing vitamin C and calcium. Dairy products are calcium-rich foods, so you might eat more of these.

Alcohol and smoking

I can't tell you anything about these and their possible effects on the prostate gland as I am teetotal and try to stay away from the bad habits. Anyway, you'll already know what doctors have forever advised us about the two, won't you.

Other things to consider

You may want to 'teach' yourself to empty your bladder just before bedtime, as this could help you get a good night's sleep. This now has also been my daily routine. And obviously, don't drink too much fluid before going to bed.

While trying to do your poo in the toilet, don't push it too hard, as this could leave you with an uncomfortable feeling for hours afterwards. To make it easier next time, try eating more foods rich in fibre so that your poo passes more smoothly – plums, or plum juice especially, can do you good whenever you're constipated.

Conclusion

That's it. All the important stuff I feel you should be aware of. Please make best friends with your prostate before it turns its back on you and you start treating it as your fiercest enemy. I must admit I made a complete mess of it all. I neglected it to the point that I didn't actually think it was there. Now I'm just a man full of regret. I really don't want you to become the same. Start acting at once so that you spare yourself the trouble and you won't experience what I have at the age of 38. My, I now assume, never-ending journey will go on until there is an ultimate cure for any problems that you and your prostate can be faced with. Good luck, mate, on your personal journey.

Please feel free to leave your feedback. Your opinion could be of great value to other people also affected by the condition. Thank you.

www.ingramcontent.com/pod-product-compliance
Lightning Source LLC
Chambersburg PA
CBHW020135180726
47992CB00023B/3161